Tips on Surviving a Brain Aneurysm

For survivors, caregivers, and loved ones

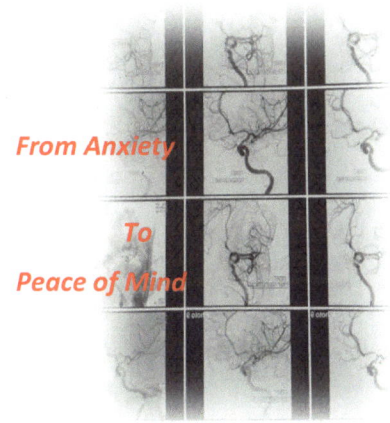

From Anxiety

To

Peace of Mind

Veronica J. Field

Dedication

I would like to dedicate this book to the following:

- ❖ My husband, Jason: Thank you honey for your pure love, dedication, commitment, and patience. I smile because you warm my heart and let me know that everything is possible as long as I believe.

- ❖ My children, Zebulon and Zalia: Thank you for giving me a reason to always look forward to tomorrow. You truly know how to brighten my day.

- ❖ My entire family: Thank you for your prayers, support, and unconditional love. You give me a complete sense of belonging.

- ❖ My fellow brain aneurysm survivors: Thank you for your bravery and endurance. We are alive for a reason.

- All the caretakers and healthcare providers: Thank you for all you do and for having such a profound level of love and patience.
- God: Thank you for the gift of life and for giving us the strength we need to endure life's challenges.

CONTENTS

FAMILIARIZE

Tips on Surviving a Brain Aneurysm for Survivors, Caregivers, and Loved Ones

The Roots

Friday, July 28th 2017 was a day like no other. I went to bed as usual but I did not wake up in the same bed. I woke up 4 days later (the days in between have been blocked out of my memory) lying in bed with all different kinds of tubes around me in the ICU unit of Netcare Unitas Hospital, Centurion, South Africa. It was on that hazy morning when I started to learn that I had suffered a brain aneurysm and had underwent a successful coiling procedure to stop the bleeding. My life has not been the same from that day. Everything changed. The real challenge for me that actually inspired me to write this book, did not start until after I received complete healing. That was about 2 months following our relocation back to the United States. I had to find a way to deal with my self-imposed fear. Fear of dying while still living. My efforts to find what I was searching for proved to be unsuccessful. When I could not find a support group close to me, I started my own blog to engage more people from across the globe by openly talking about brain aneurysms referencing to my own experience. I had to put my fears out in the open. The blog has helped me come a long way from feeling helpless to feeling helpful, from not knowing to becoming an expert in my own world. This passion and curiosity has led me to writing this book, *Tips on Surviving Brain Aneurysm- for Survivors, Caregivers, and loved ones*, which provides people with all the basic information they need to give them a peace of mind. I hope that you find this quick guide beneficial. Please note that all the material contained in this book is for informational purposes only. It should not, under no circumstances, be used to replace professional medical advice.

Section I

FAMILIARIZE

What is a brain aneurysm?

It is a bulge or ballooning in a blood vessel in the brain that occurs when a weak spot in the brain's arterial wall bulges and fills with blood (Mayo Clinic Staff)[1].

What other Terms do we use to call a Brain Aneurysm?

Intracranial aneurysm, cerebral aneurysm or berry aneurysm (Brain Aneurysm Foundation)[2].

---

[1] Mayo Clinic Staff. Brain aneurysm care at Mayo Clinic: Accessed From:

https://www.mayoclinic.org/diseases-conditions/brain-aneurysm/symptoms-causes/syc20361483

[2] Brain Aneurysm Foundation. About Brain Aneurysms. Accessed From:

https://bafound.org/about-brain-aneurysms/

Is Brain Aneurysm Life-Threatening?

It is a potentially life-threatening condition that can affect a person at any age. If a brain aneurysm ruptures, it's an emergency that can result in a stroke, brain damage, and even death if not addressed immediately.

Do all Aneurysms Rupture?

No. About 1 in 50 people in the United States have aneurysms that haven't ruptured. Approximately 50 to 80% of all aneurysms never rupture in a person's lifetime. In those that rupture, which is only about 30,000 of people in the United States per year, 40% are fatal. Of those who survive, about 66% suffer some permanent neurological deficit (Brain Aneurysm Foundation)[3].

---

[3] Brain Aneurysm Foundation. Statics and Facts. Accessed From: https://bafound.org/aboutbrain-

· aneurysms/brain-aneurysm-basics/brain-aneurysm-statistics-and-facts/

How does it look like?

It often looks like a berry hanging on a stem, giving it the nickname "berry aneurysm."

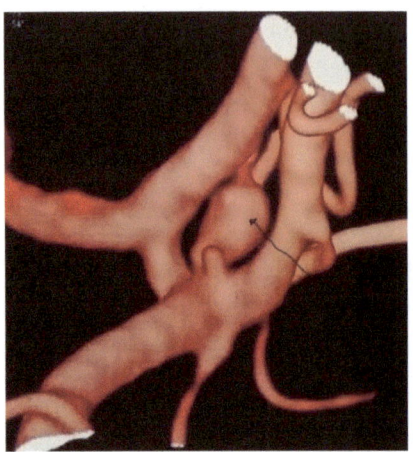

How are Brain Aneurysms Classified?

They are classified based on their type and size.

Type

There are three types of brain aneurysms:

- **Saccular aneurysm.** A saccular aneurysm is a rounded sac containing blood that is attached to the main artery or one of its branches. Also known as a berry aneurysm (because it resembles a berry hanging from a vine), this is the most common form of cerebral aneurysm. It is typically found on arteries at the base of the brain. Saccular aneurysms occur most often in adults and are found in about 2 to 3 percent of the population (National Institute of Neurological Disorders and Stroke) (Sharecare.com)[4].

- **Fusiform aneurysm**. A fusiform aneurysm balloons or bulges out on all sides of the artery.
- **Mycotic aneurysm**. A mycotic aneurysm occurs as a result of an infection that can sometimes affect the arteries in the brain. The infection weakens the artery wall, causing a bulging aneurysm to form.

Size

Aneurysms are also classified by size: small, large, and giant.

---

[4] National Institute of Neurological Disorders and Stroke. Disorder Patient-Caregiver Education

Fact Sheet Cerebral. Accessed From: https://www.ninds.nih.gov/Disorders/Patient-

Caregiver-Education/Fact-Sheets/Cerebral

- *Small aneurysms* are less than 11 millimeters in diameter (about the size of a large pencil eraser).

- *Large aneurysms* are 11 to 25 millimeters (about the width of a dime).

- *Giant aneurysms* are greater than 25 millimeters in diameter (more than the width of a quarter) (Sharecare.com)[5].

What are the Causes/Risk Factors of a Brain Aneurysm?

Major inherited risk factors for developing a brain aneurysm include:

- Genetic connective tissue disorders that weaken artery walls

- Polycystic kidney disease (in which numerous cysts form in the kidneys)

- Arteriovenous malformations (snarled tangles of arteries and veins in the brain that disrupt blood

---

[5] Sharecare. Com. How are brain aneurysms classified. Accessed on March, 2019 from:

https://www.sharecare.com/health/brain-aneurysms/how-brain-aneurysms-classified

flow. Some AVMs develop sporadically, or on their own.)

- History of an aneurysm in a first-degree family member (child, sibling, or parent)

(Sharecare.com)[6].

Other risk factors that develop over time include:

- Untreated high blood pressure

- Cigarette smoking

- Drug abuse, especially cocaine or amphetamines, which raise blood pressure to dangerous levels. Intravenous drug abuse is a cause of infectious mycotic aneurysms.

- Over age 40.

Less common risk factors include:

- Head trauma

- Brain tumor

---

[6] Ibid 1

- Infection in the arterial wall (mycotic aneurysm).

Additionally, high blood pressure, cigarette smoking, diabetes, and high cholesterol puts one at risk of atherosclerosis (a blood vessel disease in which fats build up on the inside of artery walls), which can increase the risk of developing a fusiform aneurysm (National Institute of Neurological Disorders and Stroke)[7].

Risk Factors for An Aneurysm to Rupture Include:

Smoking. Smoking is linked to both the development and rupture of cerebral aneurysms.

Smoking may even cause multiple aneurysms to form in the brain.

---

[7] National Institute of Neurological Disorders and Stroke. Disorder Patient-Caregiver Education

Fact Sheet Cerebral. Accessed From: https://www.ninds.nih.gov/Disorders/Patient-

Caregiver-Education/Fact-Sheets/Cerebral

High blood pressure. High blood pressure damages and weakens arteries, making them more likely to form and to rupture (Kleinloog, Rachel, et al. 431)[8].

Size. The most massive aneurysms are the ones most likely to rupture in a person who previously did not show symptoms.

Location. Aneurysms located on the posterior communicating arteries (a pair of arteries in the back part of the brain) and possibly those on the anterior communicating artery (a single artery in the front of the brain) have a higher risk of rupturing than those at other locations in the brain (Kleinloog, Rachel, et al.440)[9].

---

[8] Kleinloog, Rachel, et al. "Risk factors for intracranial aneurysm rupture: a systematic review." *Neurosurgery* 82.4 (2017): 431-440.

[9] Ibid 1

Growth. Aneurysms that grow, even if they are small, are at increased risk of rupture.

Family history. A family history of aneurysm rupture suggests a higher risk of rupture for aneurysms detected in family members. The most significant risk occurs in individuals with multiple aneurysms who have already suffered a previous rupture or sentinel bleed (Sharecare.com)[10].

What are the Symptoms of a Brain Aneurysm (Ruptured and Unruptured)?

Ruptured brain aneurysms usually cause bleeding into the space around the brain, called a subarachnoid hemorrhage (SAH) which can cause sudden symptoms. If you experience any or all of the following symptoms of a ruptured aneurysm, CALL 911. Things tend to deteriorate within minutes, and that is why you will need emergency responders.

---

[10] Ibid 2

- Sudden and severe headache, often described as "the worst headache of my life."
- Nausea/vomiting

- Stiff neck

- Blurred or double vision

- Sensitivity to light

- Seizure

- Drooping eyelid

- A dilated pupil

- Pain above and behind the eye

- Loss of consciousness

- Confusion

- Weakness or numbness (Lin, Ning, et al. 69)[11].

---

[11] Lin, Ning, et al. "Treatment of ruptured and unruptured cerebral aneurysms in the USA: a paradigm shift." *Journal of neurointerventional surgery* 10.Suppl 1 (2018): i69-i76.

Unruptured brain aneurysms usually have no symptoms. Typically, these aneurysms are small. Many unruptured aneurysms are found incidentally when tests are being done to screen for other conditions. Rarely, unruptured aneurysms may become large and press on nerves in the brain, causing symptoms. If you experience these symptoms, seek prompt medical attention. *Unruptured aneurysms rarely cause*:

- Blurred or double vision
- Chronic headaches
- A drooping eyelid
- A dilated pupil
- Pain above and behind one eye
- Weakness and/or numbness (Skodvin, Torbjørn Øygard, et al.880)[12].

---

[12] Skodvin, Torbjørn Øygard, et al. "Cerebral aneurysm morphology before and after rupture:

nationwide case series of 29 aneurysms." *Stroke* 48.4 (2017): 880-886.

How is a Brain Aneurysm Diagnosed?

A brain aneurysm is usually diagnosed using an MRI scan (typically in unruptured aneurysms) and angiography (MRA), or a CT scan (typically in ruptured aneurysms) and angiography (CTA). In rare cases where the ruptured aneurysm was not picked up by the CT scan, a lumbar puncture will be done to analyze for bleeding of cerebrospinal fluid (NHS)[13].

What are the Treatment Options (Ruptured and Unruptured)?

Brain aneurysms are usually treated using a variety of methods, or a combination of methods, depending on the type of aneurysm and the individual patient. These include:

1.   Microsurgical clipping

2.   Endovascular techniques:

---

[13] NHS. Diagnosis Brain Aneurysm. Accessed From:

https://www.nhs.uk/conditions/brainaneurysm/diagnosis/

- Endovascular Coiling

- Endovascular stent coiling

- Artery occlusion and bypass

- Flow diversion with stents

3. Tubular retractor system
4. Observation for unruptured aneurysms (Johns Hopkins Medicine)[14].

What are the Complications of a Brain Aneurysm?

After an aneurysm has ruptured, it may cause serious difficulties such as:

Rebleeding. Once it has ruptured, an aneurysm may rupture again before it is treated, leading to further bleeding into the brain, and causing more damage or death.

---

[14] Johns Hopkins Medicine. Neurology and Neurosurgery. Accessed From:

https://www.hopkinsmedicine.org/neurology_neurosurgery/centers_clinics/aneurysm/trea tment/index.html

Change in sodium level. Bleeding in the brain can disrupt the balance of sodium in the blood supply and cause swelling in brain cells. This can result in permanent brain damage.

Hydrocephalus. Subarachnoid hemorrhage can cause hydrocephalus. Hydrocephalus is a buildup of too much cerebrospinal fluid in the brain, which causes pressure that can lead to permanent brain damage or death. Hydrocephalus frequently occurs after subarachnoid hemorrhage because the blood blocks the normal flow of cerebrospinal fluid. If left untreated, increased pressure inside the head can cause coma or death.

Vasospasm. This frequently occurs after subarachnoid hemorrhage when the bleeding causes the arteries in the brain to contract and limit blood flow to vital areas of the brain. This can cause strokes from a lack of adequate blood flow to parts of the brain.

Seizures. Aneurysm bleeding can cause seizures (convulsions), either at the time of bleed or in the immediate aftermath. While most seizures are evident, on occasion, they may only be seen by sophisticated brain testing. Untreated seizures or those that do not respond to treatment can cause brain damage (National Institute of Neurological Disorders and Stroke)[15].

---

[15] National Institute of Neurological Disorders and Stroke. Disorder Patient-Caregiver Education

Fact Sheet Cerebral. Accessed From:

https://www.ninds.nih.gov/Disorders/PatientCaregiver-Education/Fact-Sheets/Cerebral

How long does it take to recover from a Treated Aneurysm?

Recovery is a lifelong process and varies from person to person. Active recovery can take anywhere from 2- 12 weeks including the amount of time spent in the hospital. You might need routine tests to monitor the treated aneurysm or any other aneurysms that are still intact or forming. As recovery continues, you will experience several changes such as: emotional, physical, social, and mental. You might experience stages in the recovery process that mimic the five stages of grief: denial, anger, bargaining, depression, and acceptance (The 5 Stages of Grief)[16]. It is normal. Take it one day at a time.

---

[16] GRIEF.com. THE 5 STAGES OF GRIEF. Accessed on 18 April, 2019 from:

https://grief.com/the-five-stages-of-grief/

Will my Life be the same after Treatment and Recovery?

It will take time to go back to doing the things you used to do before the rupture but you will learn to adjust with time. Take it slow but steady. Know when to stop and take a break.

What are the Chances of a Recurrence?

While most healthcare professionals will tell you that the chances of a recurrence are almost zero, it is good to be proactive and understand your body. Have routine follow-ups to manage any underlying factors such as high blood pressure and do regular scans to monitor any treated and/or unruptured aneurysms. Adopt a healthy lifestyle and try to make modifications to reduce stress.

Tips on Surviving a Brain Aneurysm

1. **Be curious about your family history**. No matter how old you are, it helps to learn about the members of your family, both immediate and extended, and any underlying health issues they might have. That will enable you to become familiar with those conditions and assess yourself if you might be at risk. Even though family history does not always pose a risk to an individual, it does not hurt to educate yourself. For my case, I have no family history of the brain aneurysm.

2.   Get a primary care physician. Most people who consider themselves "healthy" do not see the need to have a primary care physician. The reasoning behind it is that why do you need to go and look for problems if none exists. The fact is, many lives are saved through those physical assessments and preventative care measures. So, get a primary care physician and talk to him or her about your family history and any health concerns that you might have. Remember to keep up with your dental appointments as well.

3.   Know basic CPR (cardiopulmonary resuscitation). Knowing what to do especially in the initial stages when you are caught in an emergency scenario can save a life or help reduce the severity of potential adverse effects during and after treatment. The American Heart Association and The Red Cross are the most common organizations that offer CPR training classes for both caregivers and healthcare providers. I would encourage you and your family members, including children above the age of 5 years old, to take a CPR course for caregivers. I tend to think that if my husband had not known how to perform CPR, my story would have been different right now. I became unconscious in less than 3 minutes of me requesting him to give me an aspirin and having taken it. Everything was happening so fast. I started to vomit while at the same time biting on my tongue. That was a perfect scenario that could have easily led to aspiration. With his CPR knowledge, he knew exactly what to do. That was to either keep me in an upright position or side-lying while keeping the airway open.

4.   Familiarize yourself with your surroundings.
Get to know the closest hospital near your residence and the fastest way to get there. This applies to residents and visitors. When we moved to Kampala, Uganda, we spend the first month just trying to

familiarize ourselves with the hospitals in the area and the level of care they provided. Knowing the quality and level of care hospitals near you provide is especially important if you are living overseas and particularly in the developing countries. When an emergency hits, time is of an essence.

5.   **Have an emergency response system plan in place.** Knowing what to do when you find yourself in an emergency scenario can help save you a lot of time and give you a peace of mind. Everybody in your household must know your country of residence emergency phone number. In most countries, it is a three digit number. When we lived in Uganda, we had taught our 3year old how to do the radio checks and he was comfortable with it. Call a friend, a neighbor, a family member, or a coworker and let them know of your situation and current plans so they can check on you since you can't tell how fast things might change.

6. **Listen to your guts**. This is the most important tip of them all. When you start having symptoms and you kind of suspect that something is not right with your body, do not stop and play the waiting game. It is better to seek medical help and let them not find anything wrong with you than to wait for things to get worse. If you are a caregiver, seek immediate help if you think something is not normal with your loved one.

7. **Taking an Aspirin is optional. Always consult with your medical provider if you are unsure. Weigh the risks versus the benefits.** The use of aspirin has been a controversial conversation and remains a personal choice following proper counselling from a medical provider. Aspirin is an anticoagulant, and from a personal standpoint, if you have a ruptured brain aneurysm, the risk of developing a stroke or a blood clot in the brain that can possibly lead to severe brain damage is high. Taking an aspirin (only if you are the right candidate) when you initially suspect that you have a ruptured brain aneurysm, from my personal view, can help decrease the chances of developing a stroke and/or severe brain damage. Some doctors have told me that when I took that aspirin when I started feeling that something was wrong with me, helped me gain full recovery with no complications whatsoever. Some have remained neutral about the benefits of it. In the end, it all falls back to benefit versus risk.

8.   **Take one day at a time during recovery**. If you are blessed enough to make it to recovery, which I hope you or your loved one makes it, take it slow. Do not push yourself too hard. Remember that we are all different and we heal at different rates. Try to think positive and do not put so much blame on yourself for things that you had no control over. The fact that you are alive should give you a reason to be curious enough

to see what tomorrow has in store for you. God has a special purpose for you. He chose you to bear that burden because He saw something in you that qualified you for that responsibility. Do not feel depressed if you are unable to do the things that you used to do before or if your memory is not as sharp as before. Give it time and do some memory exercises. One thing you must remember is that healing begins from within. When your soul is healed, your body will surely heal.

If you are a caregiver, please be patient with your loved one. Bear in mind that recovery is probably harder for patients compared to the treatment. When your loved one realizes that he or she can't do the things they used to do before or just the thought of how life has changed for them and those around them, they feel like a burden to you. You are the only person to reassure them and give them hope when all seems to have been lost. Most patients will suffer from at least one form of depression and will lack interest in doing most things in life. It is okay and normal. Take it slow and be patient. Things will improve with time. Know when to ask for help, do not allow yourself to reach the burnout point.

If you are a caregiver and have lost a loved one due to a brain aneurysm, do not be consumed by stress. You had no control over what happened. Life is such a priceless thing, and only God can give it and take it away at His own timing. No matter how painful it is, the sad truth is that we all have a way to exit this life, and when our time comes, nothing can stop us from leaving. Pray for your loved one and know that it was their time to go and set them free.

9. **Have goals and be optimistic.** Recovery is a lifelong process, and that shouldn't discourage you from living your life to the fullest. Have goals and aim at achieving them, do not procrastinate. Take it as being granted a second chance in life, give it your very best.

Remember, life stops when you stop living and begin existing. I'm sure, if you are like me, you are more curious to know why God saved your life. Do not think too hard, enjoy your life by spreading the love. Don't forget to thank Him every day for the gift of life.

10.   **Follow-up with your doctor**. After treatment make sure you do regular follow-ups including routine testing to monitor the treated aneurysm and any unruptured or new aneurysms. The frequency of the follow-up appointments and routine testing will be determined by your medical provider. Keep up with all of your preventative care exams.

11.   **Put all of your trust unto God for He is the only one who can deliver you from any circumstance, no matter how big it is**. Do not be anxious over things you do not know or have no control over. Live your life to the fullest trusting in nothing but only in God. If you

are experiencing financial problems, talk to your doctor, church, and family members.

12.   Find a support group. You can find a support group closer to your area or find an online one. Brain aneurysm foundation usually has several support groups throughout the nation. If you can't find one close to you, then consider forming one. You can also join the Brain Aneurysm Facebook support group, I am an active member.

13.   Educate yourself by understanding the signs and symptoms. Know the different kinds of headaches and be proactive about any abnormal headaches[17].

---

[17] National Headache Foundation. The Complete Headache Chart. Accessed From:

https://headaches.org/resources/the-complete-headache-chart/

The Complete Headache Chart

Allergy Headaches

Symptoms: Generalized headache; nasal congestion; watery eyes

Precipitating Factors: Seasonal allergens, such as pollen, molds. Allergies to food are not usually a factor.

Treatment: Antihistamine medication; topical, nasal cortisone related sprays; or desensitization injections

Prevention: None

Aneurysm

Symptoms: May mimic frequent migraine or cluster headaches, caused by balloon-like weakness or bulge in blood-vessel wall. May rupture (stroke) or allow blood to leak slowly resulting in a sudden, unbearable headache, double vision, rigid neck. The individual rapidly becomes unconscious.

Precipitating Factors: Congenital tendency; extreme hypertension

Treatment: If aneurysm is discovered early, treat with surgery.

Prevention: Keep blood pressure under control to prevent.

Arthritis Headaches

Symptoms: Pain at the back of head or neck which intensifies on movement. It is caused by inflammation of the blood vessels of the head or bony changes in the structures of the neck.

Precipitating Factors: Cause of pain is unknown

Treatment: Anti-inflammatory drugs, muscle relaxants

Prevention: None

Caffeine-Withdrawal Headaches

Symptoms: Throbbing headache caused by rebound dilation of the blood vessels, occurring multiple days after consumption of large quantities of caffeine.

Precipitating Factors: Caffeine

Treatment: Treat by terminating caffeine consumption in extreme cases.

Prevention: Avoiding excess use of caffeine.

Chronic Daily Headaches

Symptoms: Refers to a broad range of headache disorders occurring more than 15 days a month; two categories are determined by duration of the headache (less than four hours and more than four hours).

Precipitating Factors: Typically evolve from transformed migraine. Although not related to chronic tension-type headache, they can evolve from episodic tension-type headache. Can be associated with medication overuse.

Treatment: Depending on the type of CHD, different treatment options exist. It is important to limit analgesic use.

Prevention: Based on diagnosis of headache, how long they last, and the number experienced per month.

Cluster Headaches

Symptoms: Excruciating pain in the vicinity of the eye; tearing of the eye; nose congestion; and flushing of the face. Pain frequently develops during sleep and may last for several hours. Attacks occur every day for weeks, or even months, then disappears for up to a year. Eighty percent of cluster patients are male, most between the ages of 20 and 50.

Precipitating Factors: Alcoholic beverages; excessive smoking

Treatment: Oxygen; ergotamine; sumatriptan; or intranasal application of local anesthetic agent

Prevention: Use of steroids; ergotamine; calcium channel blockers; and lithium

Depression and Headaches

Symptoms: People with painful organic diseased tend to become depressed.

Precipitating Factors: Causes can originate from a wide variety of complaints that can be categorized as physical, emotional, and psychic.

Treatment: The presence of depression is often subtle and the diagnosis is frequently missed. Depression is a wide spread affliction that can be treated, but first it must be unmasked.

Prevention: Physicians can prescribe tricyclic antidepressants, selective serotonin re-uptake inhibitors, or monoamine oxidize inhibitors in the treatment of headaches associated with depression.

Eyestrain Headaches

Symptoms: Usually frontal, bilateral pain directly related to eyestrain. It is a rare cause of headache.

Precipitating Factors: Muscle imbalance; uncorrected vision; astigmatism

Treatment: Correction of vision

Prevention: Correction of vision

Exertional Headaches

Symptoms: Generalized head pain of short duration (minutes to an hour) during or following physical exertion (running, jumping, or sexual intercourse), or passive exertion (sneezing, coughing, moving one's bowels, etc.)

Precipitating Factors: Ten percent caused by organic diseases (aneurysms, tumors, or blood vessel malformation). Ninety percent are related to migraine or cluster headaches.

Treatment: Cause must be accurately determined. Most commonly treated with aspiring, indomethacin, or propranolol. Extensive testing is necessary to determine the headache cause. Surgery is occasionally indicated to correct the organic disease.

Prevention: Alternative forms of exercise; avoid jarring exercises

Fever Headaches

Symptoms: Generalized head pain that develops with fever and is caused by the swelling of the blood vessels of the head.

Precipitating Factors: Caused by infection

Treatment: Aspirin; acetaminophen; NSAIDs; antibiotics

Prevention: None

Giant Cell Arteritis

Symptoms: A boring, burning, or jabbing pain caused by inflammation of the temporal arteries; pain, often around the ear, when chewing; weight loss; eyesight problems. This rarely affects people under 50.

Precipitating Factors: Cause is unknown. May be due to immune disorder.

Treatment: Steroids after diagnosis; confirmed by biopsy

Prevention: None

Hangover Headaches

Symptoms: Migraine-like symptoms of throbbing pain and nausea, but it is not localized to one side.

Precipitating Factors: Alcohol, which causes dilation and irritation of the blood vessels of the brain and surrounding tissue.

Treatment: Liquids (including broth); consumption of fructose (honey, tomato juice are a good source)

Prevention: Drink alcohol only in moderation

Hunger Headaches

Symptoms: Pain strikes just before mealtime. It is caused by muscle tension, low blood sugar, and rebound dilation of the blood vessels, oversleeping, or missing a meal.

Precipitating Factors: Strenuous dieting or skipping meals

Treatment: Regular, nourishing meals containing adequate protein and complex carbohydrates

Prevention: Regular, nourishing meals containing adequate protein and complex carbohydrates

Hypertension Headaches

Symptoms: Generalized or "hairband" type pain that is most severe in the morning. It diminishes throughout the day.

Precipitating Factors: Severe hypertension: over 200 systolic and 110 diastolic

Treatment: Treat with appropriate blood pressure medication

Prevention: Keep blood pressure under control

<u>Menstrual Headaches</u>

Symptoms: Migraine-type pain that occurs shortly before, during, or immediately after menstruation or at mid-cycle (at time of ovulation).

Precipitating Factors: Variances in estrogen levels

Treatment: At earliest onset of symptoms, treat using biodfeedback, ergotamine, dihydroergotamine, or a 5-HT agonist. Once pain has begun, treatment is identical to migraine without aura.

Prevention: Biofeedback; betablockers (propranolol, timolol); anti-convulsant (divalproex sodium); calcium blockers; and NSAIDs

Migraine with Aura

Symptoms: Warning signs develop, which may include visual disturbances or numbness in arm or leg. Warning symptoms subside within 30 minutes followed by severe pain.

Precipitating Factors: There is a hereditary component. Other factors include: Certain foods; the Pill or menopausal hormones; excessive hunger; changes in altitude; weather; lights; excessive smoking; and emotional stress.

Treatment: At earliest onset of symptoms, treat using biofeedback, ergotamine, dihydroergotamine, or a 5-HT agonist. Once pain has begun, treat with: ice packs; isometheptene; mucate; combination products containing caffeine; ergotamine; DHE injectable and nasal spray; 5-HT agonists; analgesics or medications, which constrict the blood vessels. Steroids may be helpful for prolonged attacks.

Prevention: Biofeedback; betablockers (propranolol, timolol); anti-convulsant (divalproex sodium); calcium blockers; and NSAIDs

Migraine without Aura

Symptoms: Severe, one-sided throbbing pain, often accompanied by nausea, vomiting, cold hands, sensitivity to sound and light

Precipitating Factors: There is a hereditary component. Other factors include: Certain foods; the Pill or menopausal hormones; excessive hunger; changes in altitude; weather; lights; excessive smoking; and emotional stress.

Treatment: Ice packs; isometheptene; mucate; combination products containing caffeine; ergotamine; DHE injectable and nasal spray; 5-HT agonists; analgesics or medications, which constrict the blood vessels. Steroids may be helpful for prolonged attacks.

Prevention: Biofeedback; betablockers (propranolol, timolol); anti-convulsant (divalproex sodium); calcium blockers; and NSAIDs

New Daily Persistent Headache

Symptoms: Best described as the rapid development (less than three days) of unrelenting headache. Typically presents in a person with no past history of headache.

Precipitating Factors: Does not evolve from migraine or episodic tension-type headache. It begins as a new headache and may be the result of a viral infection.

Treatment: Can resolve on its own within several months. Other cases persist and are more refractory.

Prevention: Does not respond to traditional options, but anti-seizure medications, Topamax, or Neurontine can be used.

Post-Traumatic Headaches

Symptoms: Localized or generalized pain, can mimic migraine or tension-type headache symptoms. Headaches usually occur on daily basis and are frequently resistant to treatment.

Precipitating Factors: Pain can occur after relatively minor traumas, but the cause of the pain often difficult to diagnose.

Treatment: Possible treatment by use of anti-inflammatory drugs, propranolol, or biofeedback

Prevention: Standard precautions against trauma

Sinus Headaches

Symptoms: Gnawing pain over nasal area, often increasing in severity throughout day. Pain is caused by acute infection, usually with fever, producing blockage of sinus ducts and preventing normal drainage. Sinus headaches are rare. Migraine and cluster headaches are often misdiagnosed as sinus in origin.

Precipitating Factors: Infection, nasal polyps, anatomical deformities, such as deviated septum that blocks the sinus ducts

Treatment: Treat with antibiotics, decongestants, surgical drainage, if necessary

Prevention: None

Temporomandibular Joint (TMJ) Headaches

Symptoms: A muscle-contraction type of pain, sometimes accompanied by a painful "clicking" sound on opening of the jaw. It is an infrequent cause of headache.

Precipitating Factors: Caused by malocclusion (poor bite), stress, and jaw clenching

Treatment: Relaxation, biofeedback, and the use of a bite plate are the most common treatments. In extreme cases, the correction of malocclusion may be necessary

Prevention: Same as treatment

Tension-Type Headaches

Symptoms: Dull, non-throbbing pain, frequently bilateral, associated with tightness of scalp or neck. Degree of severity remains constant.

Precipitating Factors: Emotional stress, hidden depression

Treatment: Rest; aspirin; acetaminophen; ibuprofen; naproxen sodium; combinations of analgesics with caffeine; ice packs; muscle relaxants; antidepressants, if appropriate; biofeedback; psychotherapy; temporary use of stronger prescription analgesics, if necessary.

Prevention: Avoidance of stress; use of biofeedback; relaxation techniques; or antidepressant medication

Tic Douloureux Headaches

Symptoms: Short, jab like pain in trigger areas found in the face around the mouth or jaw; frequency and longevity of pain varies. It is a relatively rare disease of the neural impulses and is more common in women after age 55.

Precipitating Factors: Cause unknown, pain from chewing, cold air, touching face. If under age 55, may result from neurological disease, such as MS.

Treatment: Anticonvulsants and muscle relaxants, neurosurgery

Prevention: None

Tumor Headache

Symptoms: Pain progressively worsens; projectile vomiting; possible visual disturbances speech or personality changes; problems with equilibrium; gait, or coordination; seizures. It is an extremely rare condition.

Precipitating Factors: The cause of tumor is usually unknown.

Treatment: If discovered early, treat with surgery or newer radiological methods.

Prevention: None

Bibliography

Brain Aneurysm Foundation. About Brain Aneurysms.

Accessed on 12 March, 2019 from:

https://bafound.org/about-brain-aneurysms/

Brain Aneurysm Foundation. Statics and Facts.

Accessed From: https://bafound.org/about-

brainaneurysms/brain-aneurysm-basics/brain-

aneurysm-statistics-and-facts/

Brain Aneurysm Foundation. Warning
Signs/Symptoms: Accessed on 17 April, 2019 from:

https://bafound.org/about-brain-

aneurysms/brain-aneurysm-basics/warning-

signssymptoms/

Grief.com THE 5 STAGES OF GRIEF. Accessed on 18
April, 2019 from:

https://grief.com/the-five-stages-of-grief/

Johns Hopkins Medicine. Neurology and
Neurosurgery. Accessed on 9 March, 2019 from:

https://www.hopkinsmedicine.org/neurology_
neurosurgery/centers_clinics/aneurysm/trea
tment/index.html

Kleinloog, Rachel, et al. "Risk factors for intracranial aneurysm rupture: a systematic review." *Neurosurgery* 82.4 (2017): 431-440.

Lin, Ning, et al. "Treatment of ruptured and unruptured cerebral aneurysms in the USA: a paradigm shift." *Journal of neurointerventional surgery* 10.Suppl 1 (2018): i69-i76.

Mayo Clinic Staff. Brain aneurysm care at Mayo Clinic: Accessed on 11 March, 2019 from:

https://www.mayoclinic.org/diseases-
conditions/brain-aneurysm/symptoms-
causes/syc-

20361483

Mayo Clinical Staff. Brain Aneurysm. Accessed on 14 March, 2019 from:

https://www.mayoclinic.org/diseases-
conditions/brain-aneurysm/symptoms-
causes/syc-

20361483

Menlo School Library. Chicago Style Guide: Accessed on 23 March, 2019 from:

https://library.menloschool.org/chicago

National Headache Foundation. The Complete

Headache Chart. Accessed in March 28 from:

https://headaches.org/resources/the-complete-

headache-chart/

National Institute of Neurological Disorders and Stroke. Disorder Patient-Caregiver Education

Fact Sheet Cerebral. Accessed on 22 March, 2019 from:

https://www.ninds.nih.gov/Disorders/Patient-Caregiver-Education/Fact-Sheets/Cerebral

NHS. Diagnosis Brain Aneurysm. Accessed on 27 April, 2019 from:

https://www.nhs.uk/conditions/brain-aneurysm/diagnosis/

Sharecare. Com. How are brain aneurysms classified.

Accessed on March, 2019 from:

https://www.sharecare.com/health/brain-

aneurysms/how-brain-aneurysms-classified

Skodvin, Torbjørn Øygard, et al. "Cerebral aneurysm morphology before and after rupture: nationwide case series of 29 aneurysms." *Stroke* 48.4 (2017): 880-886.

Your Dictionary. Example of Chicago Manual of Style Citation. Accessed on 15 April, 2019 From: https://grammar.yourdictionary.com/for-students-and-parents/example-of-chicagomanual-style-of-citation.html

www.ingramcontent.com/pod-product-compliance
Lightning Source LLC
Chambersburg PA
CBHW041109180526
45172CB00001B/179